Billie and the Brilliant Bubble
Social Distancing for Children

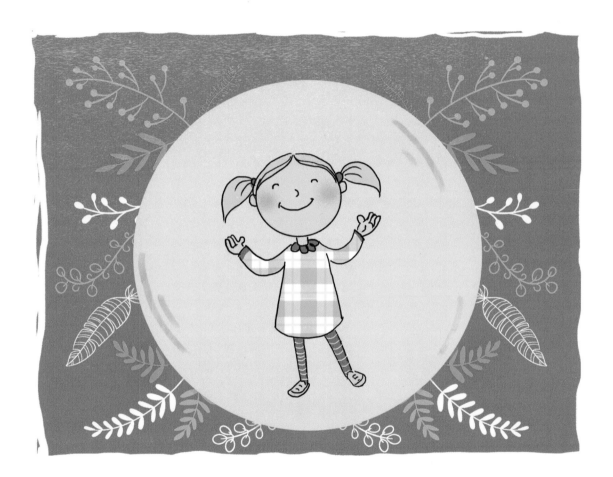

Authored by Tara Travieso
Illustrated by Bazma Ahmad

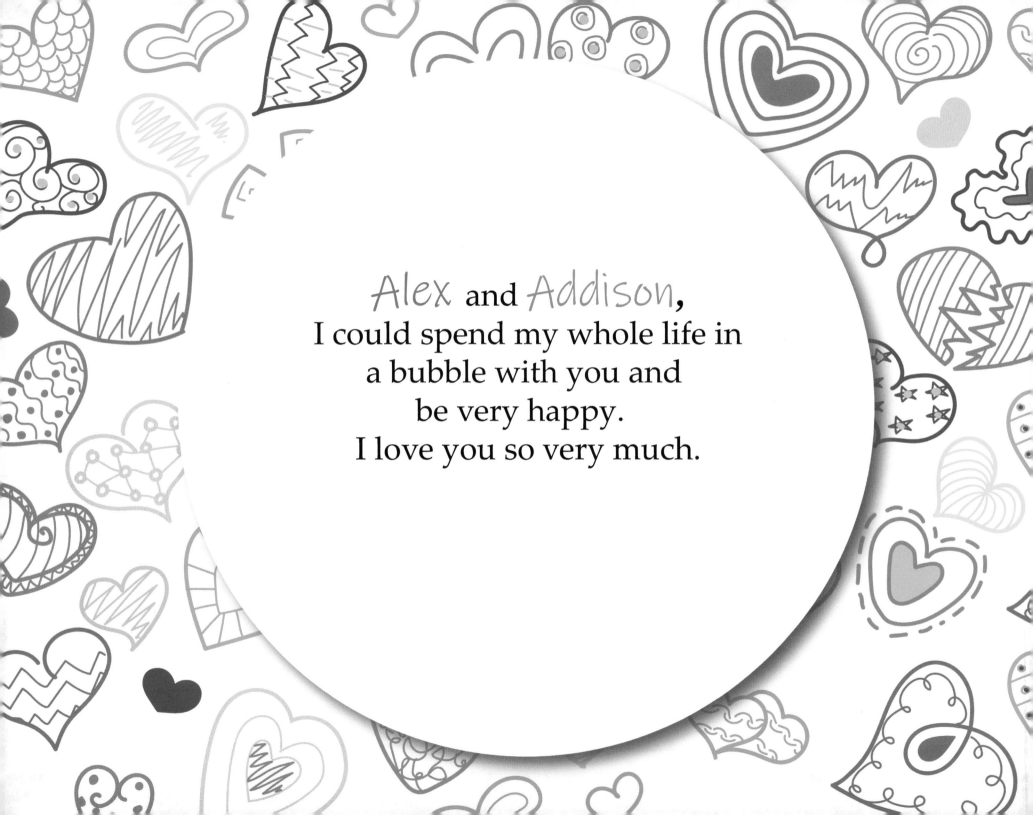

Alex and Addison,
I could spend my whole life in
a bubble with you and
be very happy.
I love you so very much.

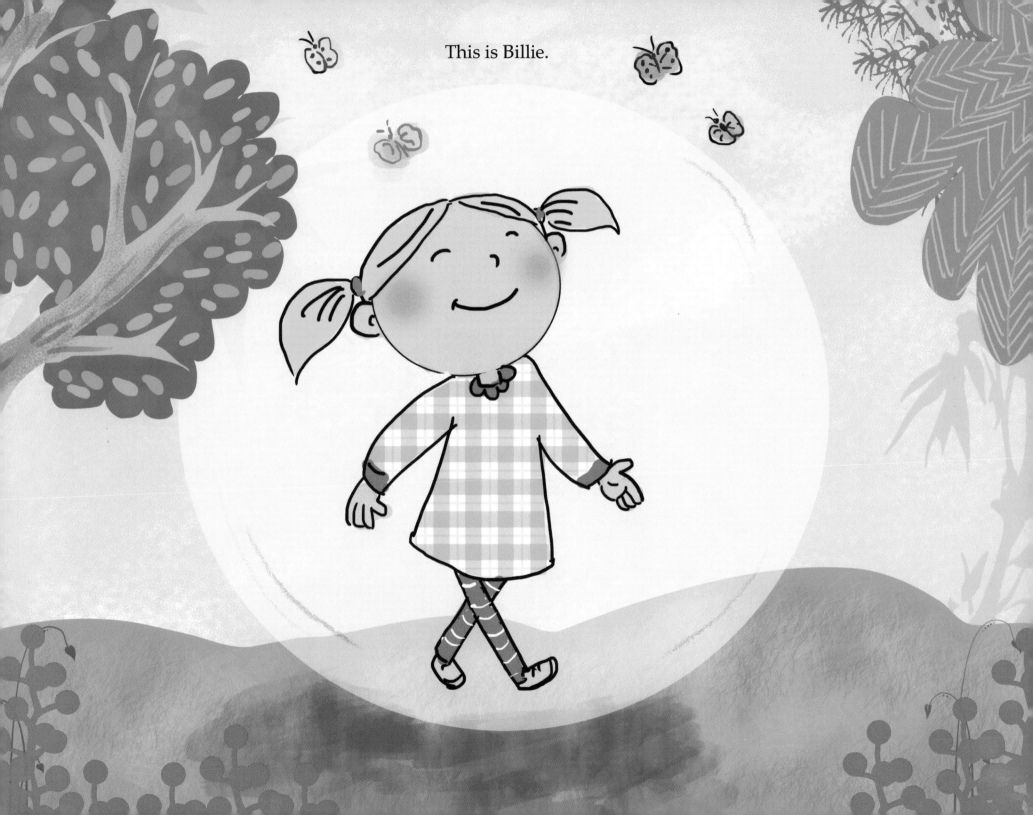

This is Billie.

One day, Billie was at her favorite place, the park, swinging as she
watched the beautiful butterflies nearby. A kickball rolled toward her.
Two children walked over to pick it up.
"Hello, I'm Billie," she said with a friendly smile.

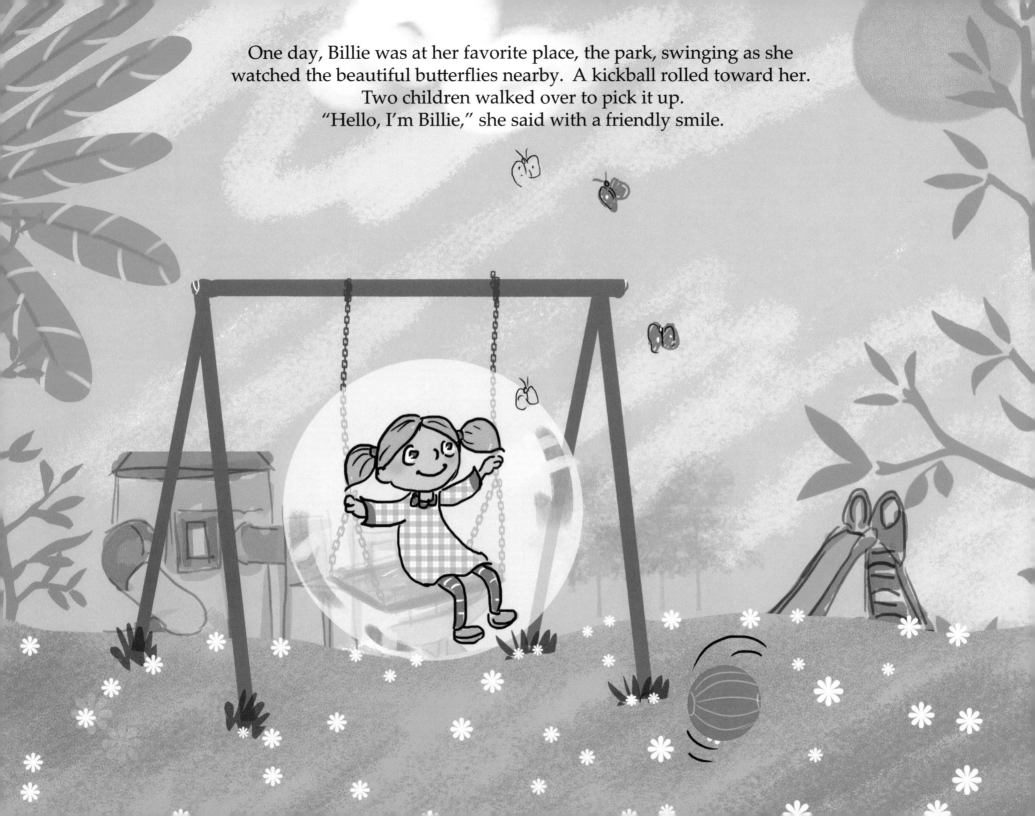

"Hi Billie, I'm Carly. And this is my brother, Cameron." Cameron continued to walk toward the ball, which continued to roll toward Billie.

"I can help you with your ball," Billie said. "Please stay there, and I will kick it to you so I don't pop my bubble."

"Bubble? What bubble?" Cameron asked curiously.

"Um, Billie, we don't see a bubble," Carly said.
"Well, technically, it's imaginary," Billie giggled. "But, it's there."

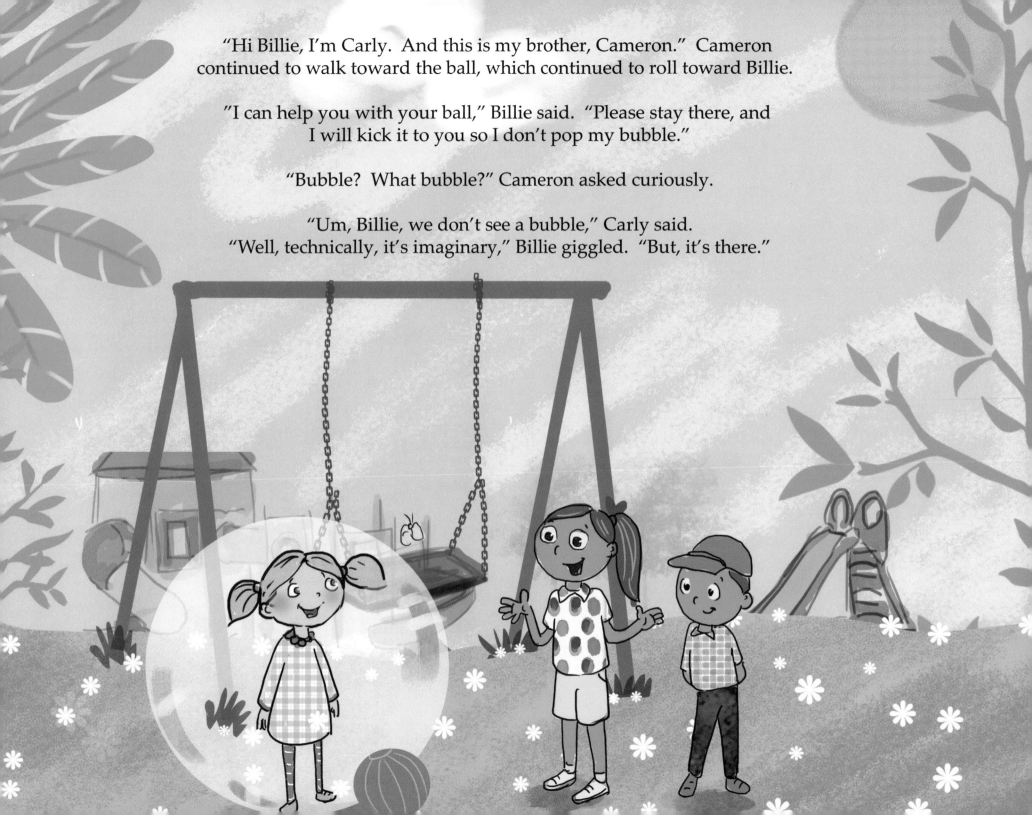

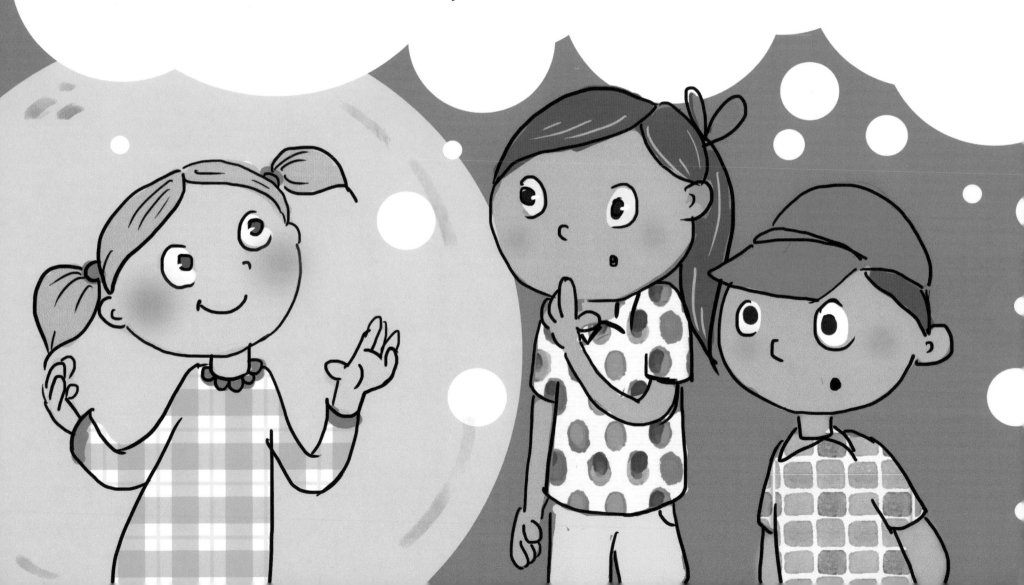

"Why do you have an imaginary bubble?" Cameron asked.

Billie happily told her new friends about her bubble. "Each morning, when I leave my house, I step into my bubble. It keeps me clean, safe, and germ-free during the day. When I go home, I step out of my bubble and wash my hands.
Do you like bubbles?"

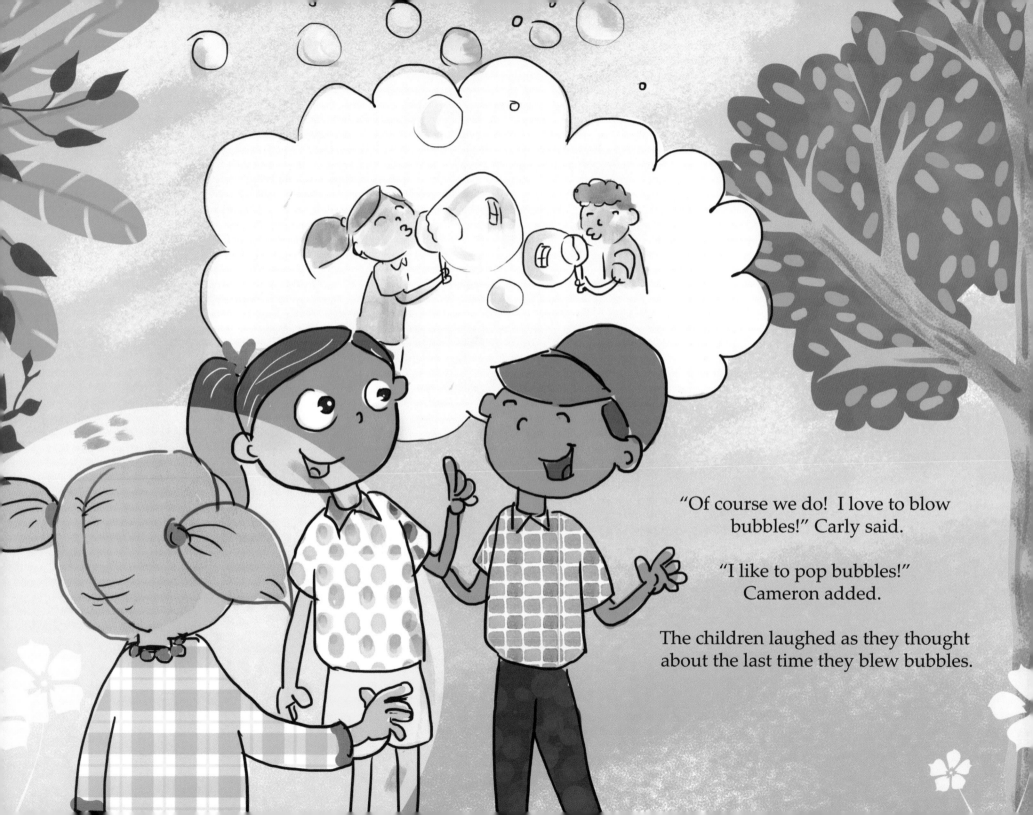

"Of course we do! I love to blow bubbles!" Carly said.

"I like to pop bubbles!" Cameron added.

The children laughed as they thought about the last time they blew bubbles.

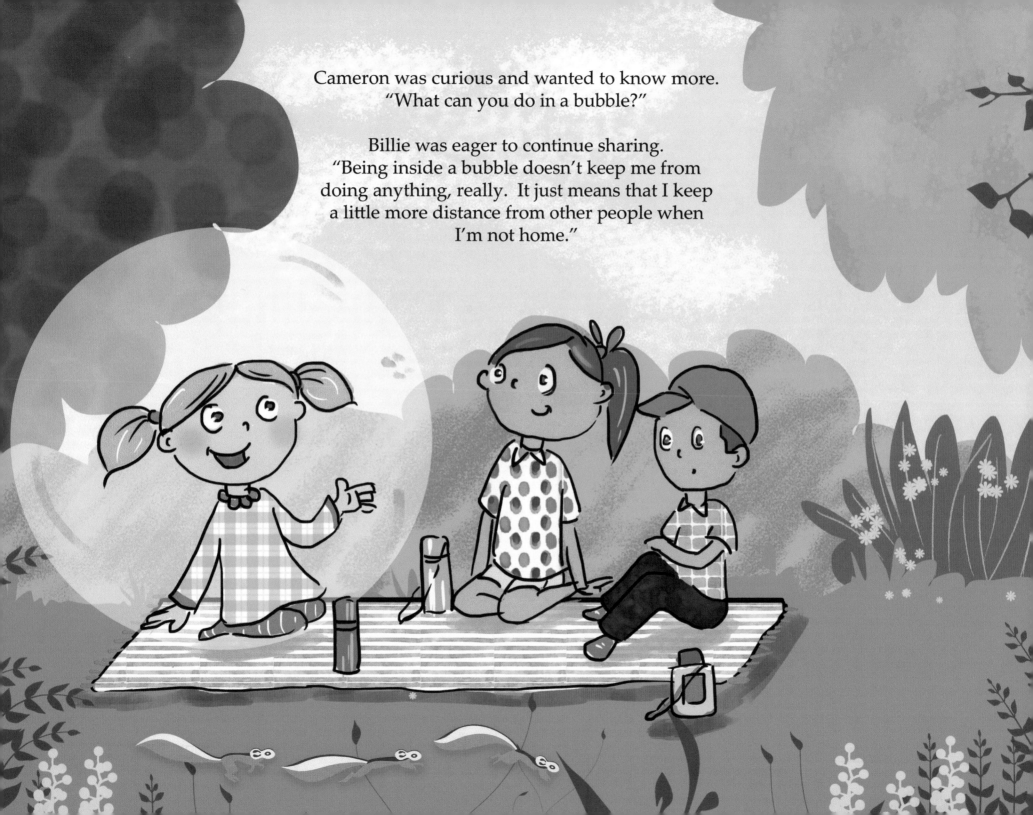

Cameron was curious and wanted to know more.
"What can you do in a bubble?"

Billie was eager to continue sharing.
"Being inside a bubble doesn't keep me from
doing anything, really. It just means that I keep
a little more distance from other people when
I'm not home."

"I can play outside."

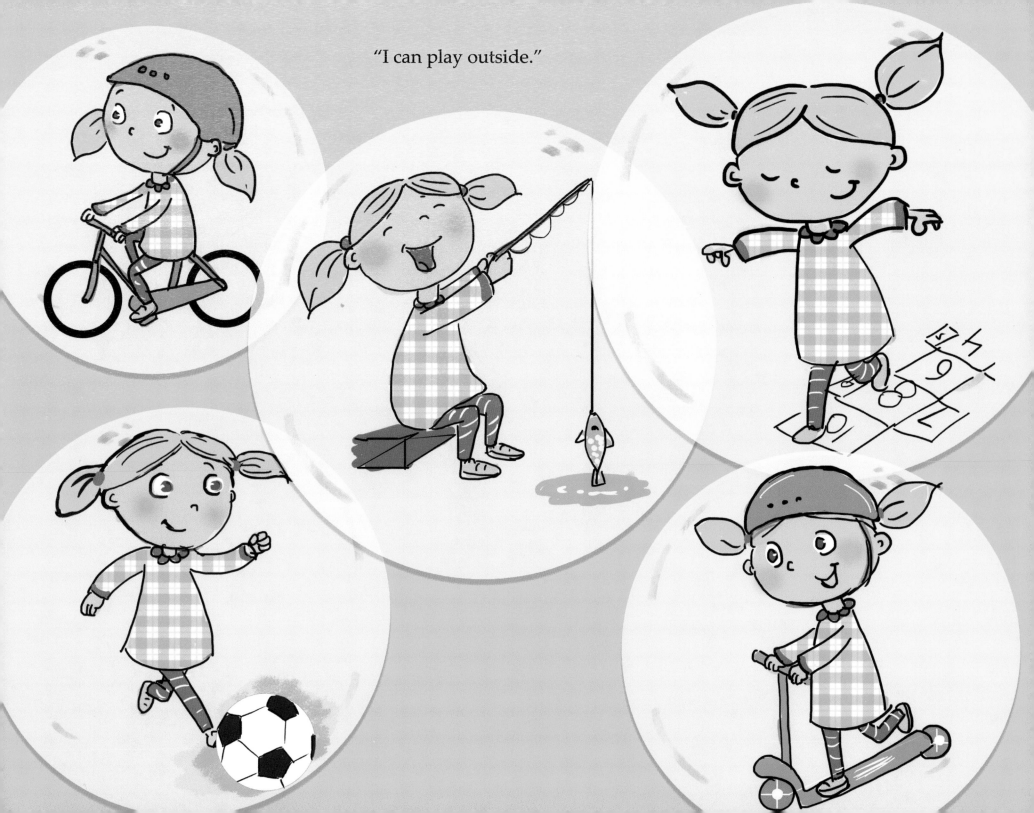

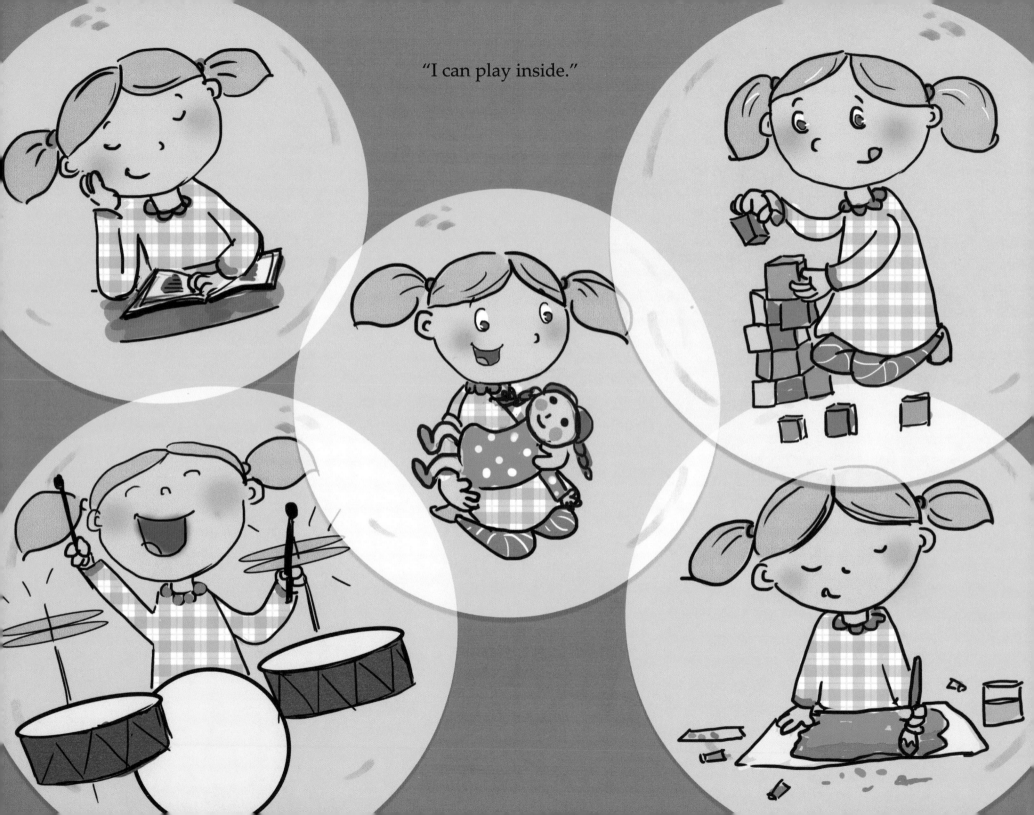

"I can play inside."

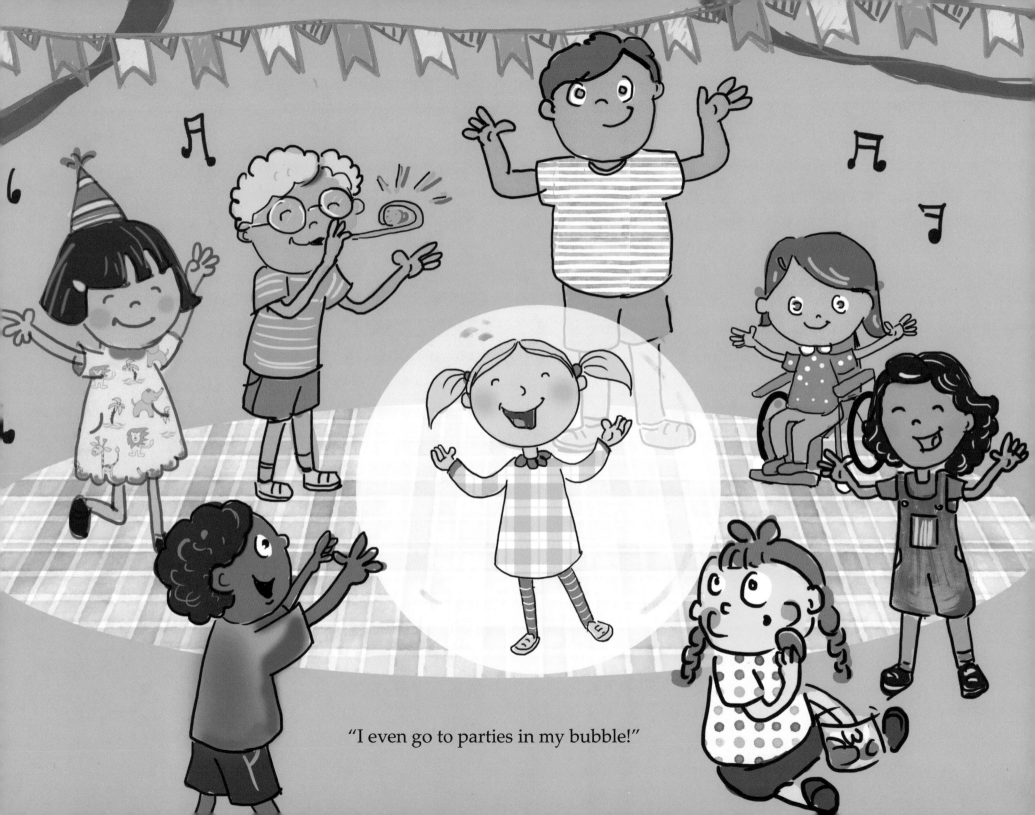

"I even go to parties in my bubble!"

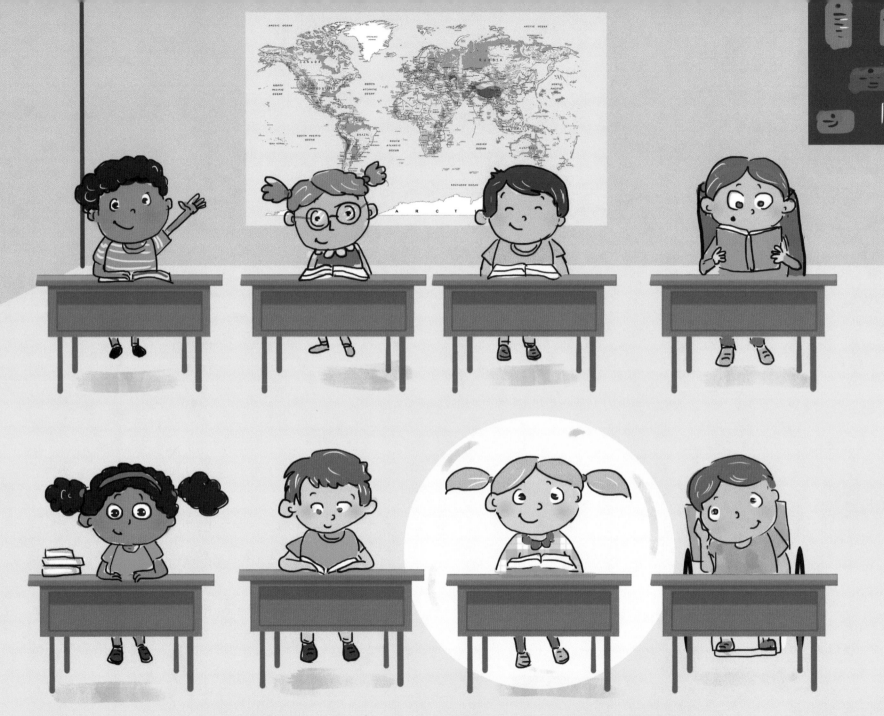

"Are you allowed to take your bubble to school?" asked Carly.

"Oh yes, I sure am. I also take it to dance lessons, restaurants, and the beach."

"Most importantly, the bubble keeps me, and all the people around me, healthy. You see, any germs that I have stay in my bubble, so I don't get anyone else sick."

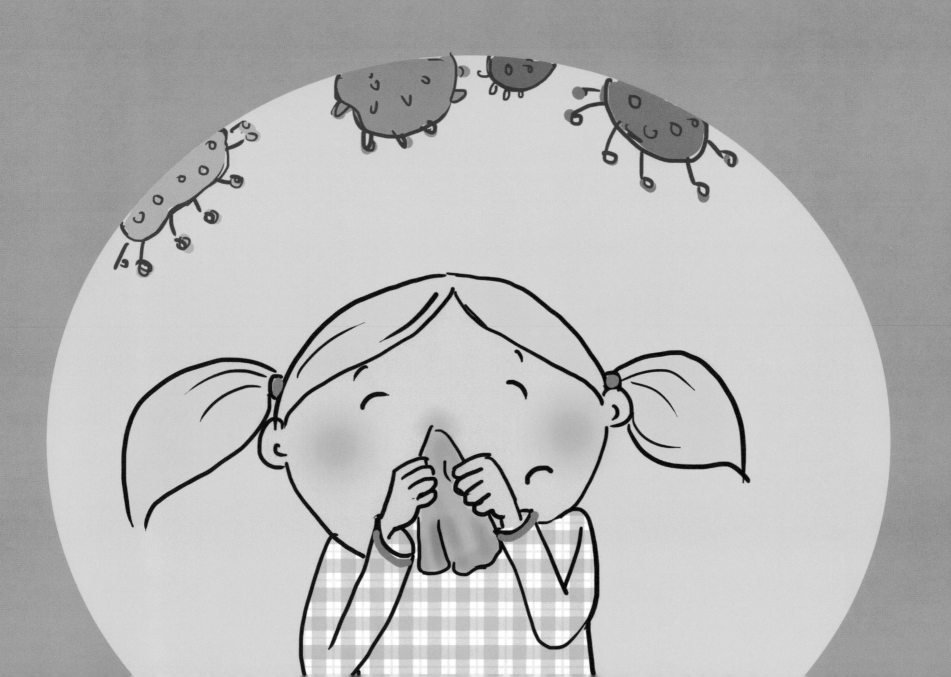

"And the germs that other people have stay outside my bubble, so they don't get me sick."

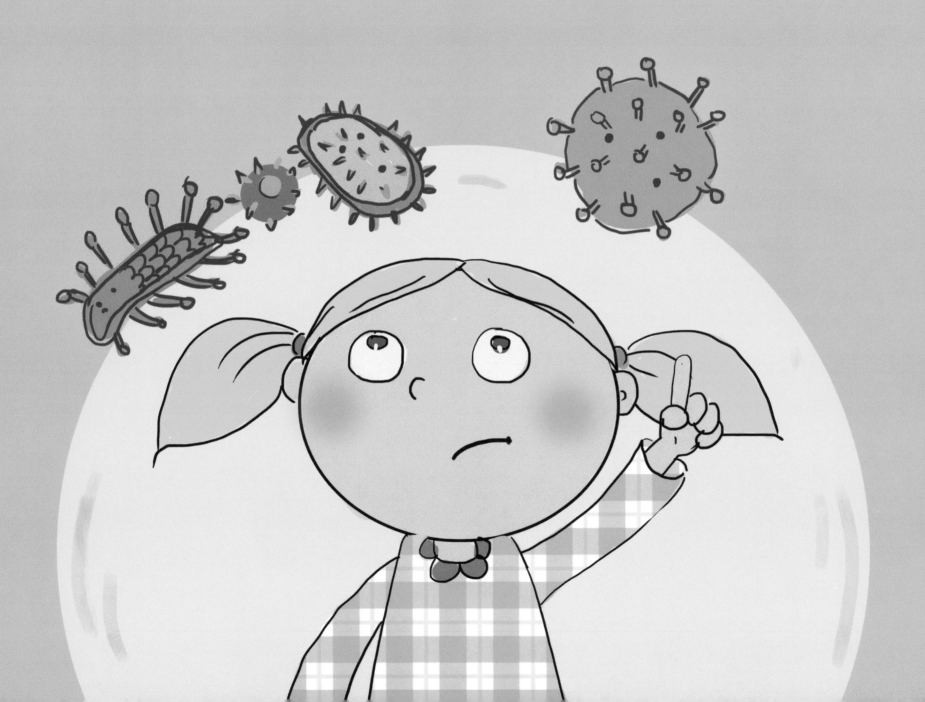

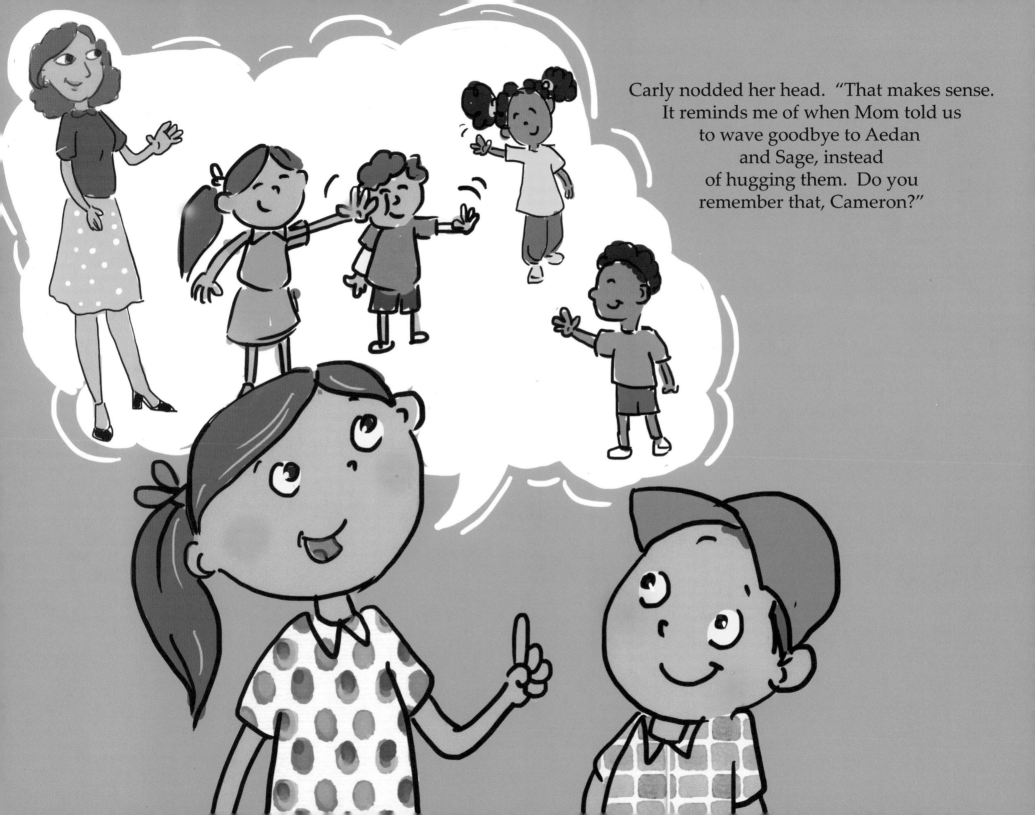

Carly nodded her head. "That makes sense. It reminds me of when Mom told us to wave goodbye to Aedan and Sage, instead of hugging them. Do you remember that, Cameron?"

"Oh yeah, that's right," Cameron replied. "Or when my teacher reminds us to stay six feet apart when we walk to the library."

He added, "Germs are yucky and make us sick. I stopped sucking my thumb, so I don't get germs in my mouth."

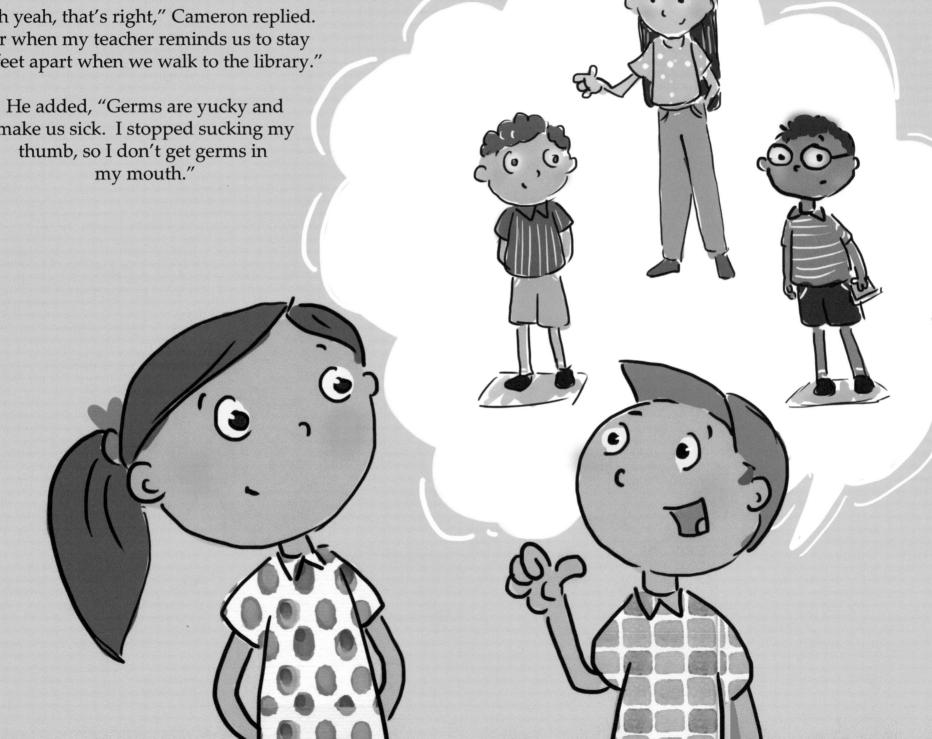

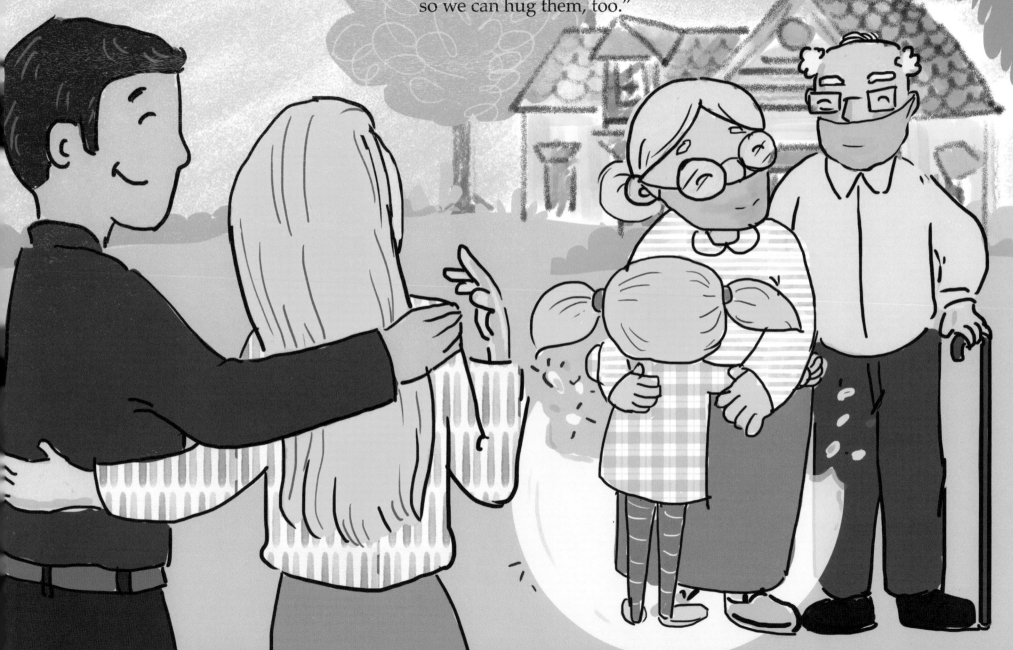

"But, don't you get sad when you can't hug your Mommy or Daddy?"

"I hug my family all the time. When we go home, we pop our bubbles and wash our hands. Then, we can safely hug each other. And, when everyone is healthy, we have Grandma and Grandpa over so we can hug them, too."

"I wish I could have a bubble," Carly whispered quietly.
"You can, Carly! My Mommy taught me how to make bubbles for other people. Would you like one?"

Carly quickly replied, "Pretty please with sugar on top!"

"I'd like one, too, please," Cameron chimed in.

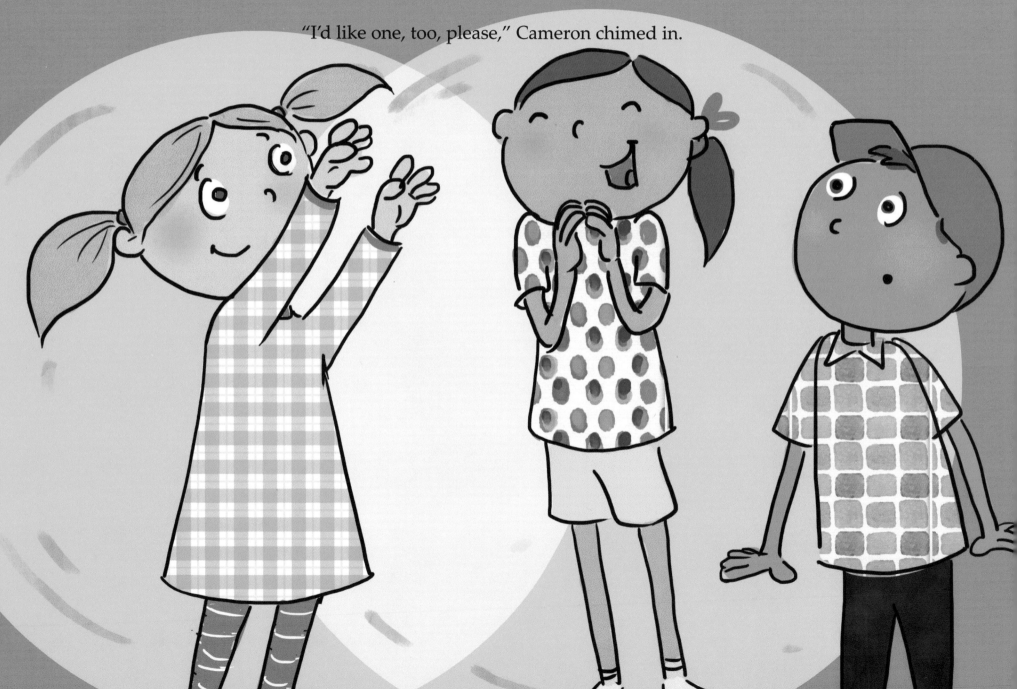

"Then, Billie zippered an imaginary zipper in front of Carly, from her head down to her toes. "Step in."
Carly stepped into the bubble, one foot at a time.

"This is fun," she said with a chuckle.

Then, it was Cameron's turn. As he stepped in, he pretended to touch the top of his new bubble.

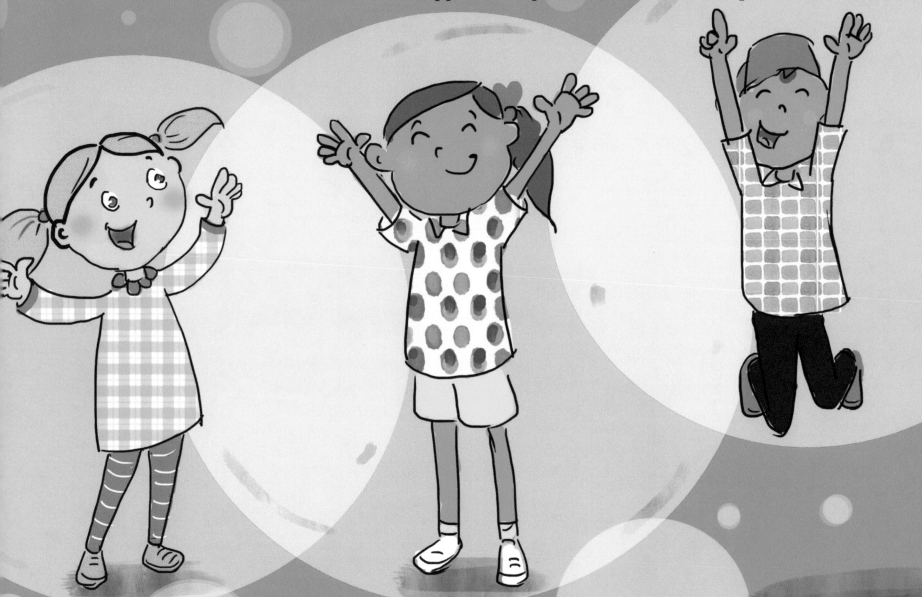

"Oh, that's my Mom calling me. I have to go now, but I hope we can play again another day," Billie said to her new friends.

"We do, too. Thank you for telling us about your imaginary bubble," Cameron said.
"Now we can stay healthy like you!"

"Billie, it's time to go, Honey Bunches!"

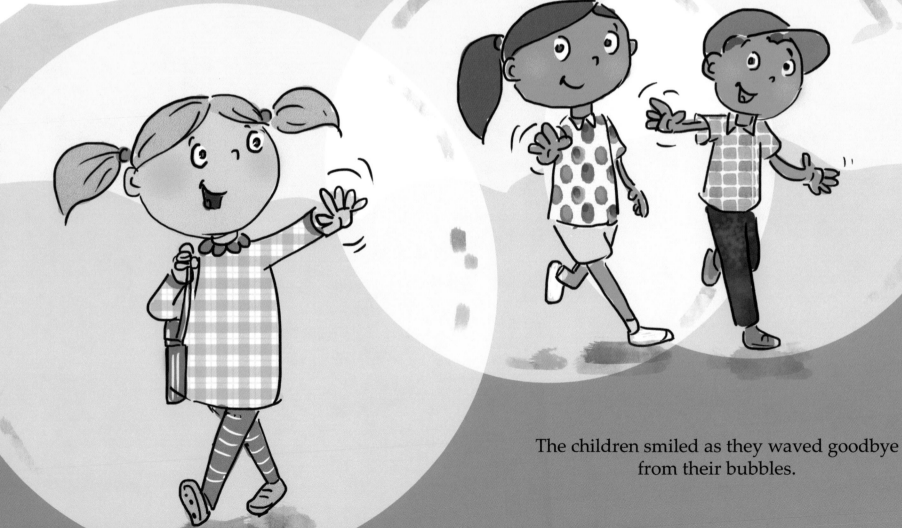

The children smiled as they waved goodbye from their bubbles.

About the Author

Tara Travieso is the proud mother of two beautiful girls, Alexandria (3) and Addison (2). Tara is married to her college sweetheart, Robert. They love to travel, enjoy good food, spend time outside, and entertain family and friends.

After living in several exciting cities around the world, including New York City, London, Washington D. C., and Miami, Tara and Robert decided to plant roots in their home state, Florida, for the next chapter of their life. They now reside in Northeast Florida, where they enjoy the lovely mix of seasons and the incredible beaches.

Shortly after their move, the COVID-19 pandemic struck. With schools closed and business travel banned, Tara spent more time at home with her family. She found the creative minds and wild imaginations of her children inspiring, energizing, and increasingly important to maintaining happiness and balance.

Thanks to the support of her family and friends, Tara considers this book a team effort and reflection of the wonderful things that we can accomplish together, even when we must be apart.

Billie and the Brilliant Bubble was born when social distancing orders began in early 2020. Tara wanted a fun and simple way to explain the new guidelines to her young daughters, Alexandria and Addison.

One day, while Tara and the girls were on a walk, it dawned on her that Alex and Addison loved bubbles. It would be fun pretending they were inside an imaginary bubble that protects them from germs and keeps their family and friends healthy. When restrictions were in place, the girls were still able to walk around the nature trail, ride their scooters, and go for ice cream with Mommy and Daddy, all in the safety of their imaginary bubbles. Alex and Addison had so much fun with their magical bubbles, Tara knew she had to share the idea.

Billie and the Brilliant Bubble simplifies the concept of social distancing to help families teach their children the importance of social distancing. Tara sincerely hopes you and your family enjoy many bubble-filled adventures of your own.

CPSIA information can be obtained at www.ICGtesting.com
Printed in the USA
LVIW011435090720
660235LV00017B/184